OCCASION
P A P E

MW00608361

A Comparison of the Health Systems in China and India

Sai Ma, Neeraj Sood

RAND CENTER FOR ASIA PACIFIC POLICY

International Programs at RAND

The research described in this report results from the RAND Corporation's continuing program of self-initiated research, which is made possible, in part, by the generous support of donors and by the independent research and development provisions of RAND's contracts for the operation of its U.S. Department of Defense federally funded research and development centers. The research was conducted within the RAND Center for Asia Pacific Policy, part of the RAND International Programs.

Library of Congress Cataloging-in-Publication Data

Ma, Sai, 1979–
   A comparison of the health systems in China and India / Sai Ma, Neeraj Sood.
     p. ; cm.
   Includes bibliographical references.
   ISBN 978-0-8330-4483-9 (pbk. : alk. paper)
   1. Medical care—China. 2. Medical care—India. 3. Medical policy—China. 4. Medical policy—India.
I. Sood, Neeraj. II. Rand Corporation. III. Title.
   [DNLM: 1. Delivery of Health Care—China. 2. Delivery of Health Care—India. 3. Cross-Cultural
Comparison—China. 4. Cross-Cultural Comparison—India. 5. Health Policy—China. 6. Health Policy—
India. 7. Patient Satisfaction—China. 8. Patient Satisfaction—India. 9. Quality of Health Care—China.
10. Quality of Health Care—India. W 84 JC6 M111c 2008]

RA395.C53M3 2008
362.10951—dc22

                                                                                           2008021840

The RAND Corporation is a nonprofit research organization providing objective analysis and effective solutions that address the challenges facing the public and private sectors around the world. RAND's publications do not necessarily reflect the opinions of its research clients and sponsors.

RAND® is a registered trademark.

Published 2008 by the RAND Corporation
1776 Main Street, P.O. Box 2138, Santa Monica, CA 90407-2138
1200 South Hayes Street, Arlington, VA 22202-5050
4570 Fifth Avenue, Suite 600, Pittsburgh, PA 15213-2665
RAND URL: http://www.rand.org/
To order RAND documents or to obtain additional information, contact
Distribution Services: Telephone: (310) 451-7002;
Fax: (310) 451-6915; Email: order@rand.org

Preface

In this paper, we compare the health systems of China and India—the world's two most populous countries, each of which is undergoing dramatic demographic, societal, and economic transformations—to determine what approaches to improving health in these two countries do and do not work. In particular, we compare the health systems of China and India along three dimensions: policy levers, intermediate outcomes, and ultimate ends. *Policy levers* are policies or behaviors that affect the financing, organization, and regulation of health care. *Intermediate outcomes* are the efficiency, quality, and level of access to care. The *ultimate ends* of a health care system are to promote better health, reduce the financial risks associated with medical care, and increase consumer satisfaction.

We conclude that both China and India have achieved substantial gains in life expectancy and disease prevention since independence; these gains are more substantial in China. However, both countries' health systems provide little protection against financial risk, and patient satisfaction is a lower priority than it should be. This paper identifies priority areas for reform in each country that can help improve the performance of each health system. Both countries must

- restructure health care financing to reduce the burden of out-of-pocket medical care costs on individual patients
- increase access to care, especially in rural areas
- reduce dependence on fee-for-service contracts that promote overutilization of medical care
- build capacity for addressing and monitoring emerging diseases
- match hospital capabilities with local needs.

The lessons learned from China and India in the past three decades will not only affect people residing in these two countries, but will also shed light on the challenges and options that other countries face.

This paper should interest health policymakers and researchers in China and India, health policy analysts who want to apply lessons learned in China and India to other developing countries, and those who are interested in economic development, social context, and individual well-being in China and India. This paper is the result of the RAND Corporation's continuing program of self-initiated independent research. Support for such research is provided, in part, by donors and by the independent research and development provisions of RAND's contracts for the operation of its U.S. Department of Defense federally funded research and development centers.

This research was conducted within RAND's Center for Asia Pacific Policy. The RAND Center for Asia Pacific Policy, part of International Programs at the RAND Corporation, aims to improve public policy by providing decisionmakers and the public with rigorous, objective research on critical policy issues affecting Asia and U.S.–Asia relations.

For more information on the RAND Center for Asia Pacific Policy, contact the Director, Bill Overholt. He can be reached by email at William_Overholt@rand.org; by phone at 310-393-0411, extension 7883; or by mail at RAND, 1776 Main Street, Santa Monica, California 90407-2138. More information about RAND is available at www.rand.org.

Contents

Figures

Tables

Acknowledgements

We would like to thank Susan Everingham and Bill Overholt, who found the funding to support this work, and Peter Hussey and Shinyin Wu, who provided constructive and thoughtful comments and suggestions on the initial draft. We would also like to thank Erin-Elizabeth Johnson, David Adamson, Lynn Rubenfeld, Mary Wrazen, and Christina Pitcher for providing excellent editorial assistance.

Abbreviations

CDC   Centers for Disease Control and Prevention

CHC   community health center

CHI   community-based health insurance scheme

CMS   Cooperative Medical System

DALY   disability adjusted life years

FFS   fee for service

GDP   gross domestic product

HMO   health maintenance organization

LBW   low birth weight

MSA   medical savings account

NHE   national health expenditure

OECD   Organisation for Economic Co-operation and Development

PHC   primary health center

PRB   Population Reference Bureau

SARS   severe acute respiratory syndrome

SC   subcenter

WHO   World Health Organization

CHAPTER ONE

Introduction

China and India have much in common. Both have rapidly developing economies and large populations. Together, their more than 2 billion residents account for one-third of the total world population. Over the past 50 years, both countries have also made substantial gains in health, including increased life expectancy, reduced infant mortality, and the eradication of several diseases. Yet, despite these gains, the health status of residents of China and India still lags that of other populations, and the health gains in each country have been uneven across subpopulations. This raises an important question: How can health in these two countries be improved? One starting point is a comparison of Chinese and Indian health systems. Although the two nations' health systems have a great deal in common, they also display fundamental differences. A comparison can illuminate the challenges that are common to both and also underscore the unique challenges each faces. Such a comparison is also timely, because health care reform is high on the political agenda of both countries and policy options are being debated. It is our hope that this analysis and the implications we draw for improvement will help inform this debate.

Analytical Framework

This paper compares the health systems of China and India. The dissimilarities, distinctions, and diversity that exist among health systems in different countries make it difficult to arrive at a universal definition of a health care system, consequently complicating cross-country comparisons. This paper adopts the definition developed by Hsiao (2003) and others (Roberts et al., 2004), which is in turn based on the conceptualization and work of other researchers: *"A health system is defined by those principal causal components that can explain the system's outcomes. These components can be utilized as policy instruments to alter the outcomes"* (Hsiao, 2003, p. 5, emphasis in original). The advantage of this definition compared with others is that it answers *why* and *how* a particular health system produces a set of outcomes. Therefore, it is a particularly useful analytical framework for comparative analysis.

Our comparison focuses on three different dimensions of the health care systems in China and India. Figure 1.1 identifies each dimension and describes its critical components. First, we analyze each country's health system policy levers.[1] The *policy levers* of the health system are structural parameters that directly or indirectly affect health and health care; those parameters

---

[1]   Hsiao and his colleagues often use the term *means* as a synonym for *policy levers*. In this paper, to avoid confusion, we use *policy levers* throughout.

Figure 1.1
Policy Levers, Intermediate Outcomes, and Ultimate Ends of a Health System

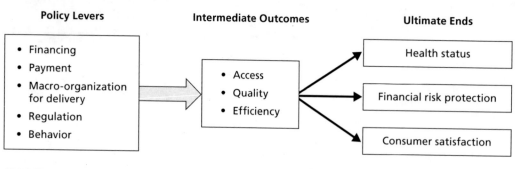

SOURCE: Hsiao, 2003.
RAND *OP212-1.1*

that cannot be altered by policies or government regulation are not included in the policy lever rubric. Culture, for example, is not a policy lever; it cannot be easily changed in the short term, although it may be an important determinant of health (Hsiao, 2003; Roberts et al., 2004). Next, we analyze *intermediate outcomes*. Important intermediate outcomes include access to health care, levels of efficiency and waste in the system, and the quality of care. Finally, we analyze how completely the health system achieves its *ultimate ends*, which include improving citizen health, providing financial protection against health risks, and improving overall consumer satisfaction with the health system.

A Demographic Overview of the Two Countries

Before we move on to disentangling the health systems of China and India, we provide a demographic overview to help foster a better understanding of some of the issues and challenges the two countries face (see Table 1.1). China and India are the two most populous countries in the world. However, their demographic profiles and trends differ dramatically. In particular, India's population is much younger and is growing at a faster rate. In 2004 India's more than 1 billion residents had a median age of 24.4 years; only 4 percent of the population was older than 64, whereas 36 percent was younger than 15. The annual population growth rate was estimated at 1.7 percent. The total dependence ratio, which compares the number of working-age individuals to nonworking-age individuals (i.e., children and the elderly), was quite high, totaling 60 per 100 persons ages 15 to 60; this means that for every 100 working residents, 60 were not working. This high ratio is primarily due to the high proportion of Indians younger than 15.

At 1.3 billion, China's population in 2004 was the largest in the world, totaling more than four times the population of the third most populous country, the Unites States. Yet population growth in China has slowed in the past decade; the annual population growth rate was only 0.8 percent between 1994 and 2004. According to a Population Reference Bureau (PRB) projection, China's population will be overtaken by India's in 2050. At the same time, the population is graying rapidly, owing both to falling fertility (the total fertility rate is 1.7)[2]

---

[2] The total fertility rate refers to the average number of children born to a woman over her lifetime.

Table 1.1
Population Indicators

Country	Population, 1994	Annual Growth Rate, 1994–2004 (%)	Dependence Ratio, 1994[a]	Dependence Ratio, 2004[a]	Fertility Rate, 1994[b]	Fertility Rate, 2004[b]	Percentage in Age Group, 2005		
							<15	15–64	>64
China	1,315,409,000	0.8	48	42	1.9	1.7	20	72	8
India	1,087,124,000	1.7	68	60	3.7	3.0	36	60	4

SOURCES: WHO, 2006; Population Reference Bureau, 2006.

[a] Per 100 persons.

[b] Per woman.

and increasing longevity (the average life expectancy is 72 years): In 2004 as much as 8 percent of the total population was older than 64, while 20 percent was younger than 15. The proportion of Chinese age 65 and over is projected to reach about 20 percent in 2040. As a result, the ratio of working-age people to elderly people will decrease from 5:1 to 3:1 (United Nations in China, n.d.).

The rest of this paper is organized as follows. In Chapter Two, we present a brief history of the health systems in China and India. The three subsequent chapters compare and analyze the two countries' health systems along three dimensions: overall current performance in achieving ultimate ends, intermediate outcomes observed, and policy levers employed. We highlight each system's strengths and weaknesses. We conclude by discussing the policy implications of addressing existing and emerging challenges and describing what China and India can learn from each others' experiences.

CHAPTER TWO

A Brief History of the Health Systems in China and India

In this chapter, we briefly review the historical, social, and political forces that shaped the health systems in China and India over the past 50 years. During that period, both countries gained independence (in the late 1940s) and increased economic and social openness (in the 1980s and 1990s). We also identify the successes achieved and lessons learned as health systems evolved in each country.

Health System Evolution in China

After the establishment of the People's Republic of China in 1949, the country was recovering from the chaos of long conflicts both internally and with Japan. As a result, Chinese health conditions had declined, with health indicators at the lowest level compared with other countries at a comparable level of development (World Bank, 1997). During this period, the ruling Communist Party espoused the typical 20th century communist ideology and believed that the people, represented by the government, should jointly own all means of production; there was no role for the private sector. Therefore, beginning in 1949, the government owned, funded, and ran all health care facilities, including large hospitals in urban areas and small township clinics in the countryside. All providers were employees of the state. Meanwhile, private health practice and private ownership of health facilities disappeared along with other private business.

In 1950, at the First National Health Work Conference, the central government announced four fundamental principles for medical and health work: service for workers, peasants, and soldiers; prevention first; combining Chinese medicine and Western medicine; and integrating "mass campaign"[1] into health care work as a core mechanism (Project Team of the Development Research Center of the State Council of China, 2005).

Because of a unique dual social and economic structure, health care was (and still is) delivered very differently in China's urban and rural areas. In the cities, all revenues and expenditures were planned and controlled by the government, health services were directly organized and almost completely funded by the government, and urban residents only paid a small "registration fee" to receive treatment. In the rural areas, the commune was the keystone of all aspects of life. Communes, the critical institutes that represented the peasants, owned the land and organized every activity, including farming, distributing products, and supplying social services such as health care and education. Health care was provided in the Cooperative Medi-

---

1 *Mass campaign* is a term directly translated from Chinese. It refers to a public campaign directed at all levels.

cal System (CMS), which was mostly financed through a commune's collective revenue and was minimally supported by the central government in the form of low-priced medicine and equipment. The CMS operated village and township health clinics that were staffed mostly by practitioners who had only basic health care training. These so-called barefoot doctors received much publicity and praise in the West for their supposed effectiveness in meeting the needs of rural populations (Blumenthal and Hsiao, 2005; Hesketh and Wei, 1997).

Although the economy grew very slowly, the Chinese health system achieved enormous improvements in health and health care between approximately 1950 and 1990: Life expectancy almost doubled (rising from 35 to 68 years), and there was a dramatic drop in infant mortality (falling from 200 to 34 per 1,000 live births) (Blumenthal and Hsiao, 2005). These improvements coincided with major investments in public health through a highly centralized governmental agency modeled on the Soviet Union's system of the early 1950s (Liu, Rao, and Fei, 1998). In particular, health care delivery was organized as a three-tier, bottom-up delivery system. At the lowest level, rural village or urban street health clinics provided basic preventive and curative care and referred patients who needed additional treatment to township or community health centers. County or district hospitals provided specialized care to the sickest patients through an extensive network of hospitals in both urban and rural areas (Project Team of the Development Research Center of the State Council of China, 2005). Additionally, special attention was paid to training health care personnel. Thousands of "village doctors" (i.e., the former barefoot doctors), were selected by county health authorities to receive three to four months of initial training as well as additional, annual training to upgrade their skills (Hsiao, 1995).

By the beginning of the 1980s, China was undergoing an epidemiological transition common in many developed countries: The prevalence of infectious diseases radically decreased, some infectious diseases (such as polio) were nearly eradicated, and chronic diseases (e.g., heart disease, cancer, and stroke) became the leading cause of illness and death (Chinese Ministry of Health, 2004). In 1984 the World Health Organization (WHO) praised China's achievement in providing everyone with primary health care.

Those improvements in health outcomes have been attributed to many factors. The government emphasized a public health approach by focusing on prevention rather than cures and on dissemination of health education and information. Both these policies are generally regarded as cost-effective approaches to improving population health.

Although the achievement in improving health and expanding health care infrastructure during the planned-economy period is certainly indisputable, the merits of this health system may have been overestimated. First, as noted, health in China was extremely poor when the country gained independence. It might have been easy to improve health starting from this low point, since several urgent needs could have been easily addressed. Second, health care is not the only factor that influences health. Between approximately 1950 and 1990, nutrition, hygiene, education, living standards, and even culture changed dramatically in China (Hsiao, 1995). These changes could have greatly affected improvements in health. Finally, while the centralized health care system may have functioned well for certain purposes, the shortcomings of the system might have been hidden by lack of information. For example, equity was not a big concern 40 years ago, partly because health care resources were scarce and rather homogenous in general, and partly because there was little information and transparency about disparities, such as high-level Communist Party cadres receiving preferred treatment in specialized hospitals.

Since the early 1980s, China has experienced fundamental economic reform and societal transformation. In this context, the health care system—and many other public services—have undergone changes that are often characterized as privatization. As early as 1980, the Chinese Ministry of Health reviewed the situation and recommended legalizing private medical practice under strict regulation. In 1985 the State Council, the Chinese equivalent of the U.S. cabinet, directed that private medical practice be encouraged (Lim, Yang, Zhang, Feng, et al., 2004).

Subsequently, decisionmakers at the national level made a number of critical decisions about partially marketing and privatizing the delivery—though not the ownership—of some health care services. First, China dramatically changed its health care financing structure, shifting a substantial share from the central government to individual consumers. Figure 2.1 shows that the central government's share of national health care spending decreased from 32 to 15 percent between 1978 and 2002, even though the absolute amount of government expenditure on health increased during this time. In the meantime, the proportion of individual out-of-pocket payments increased from 20 to 58 percent (Project Team of the Development Research Center of the State Council of China, 2005). The central government also transferred responsibility for funding health care services to provincial and local authorities through local taxation (Blumenthal and Hsiao, 2005; Hesketh and Zhu, 1997).

Second, the government imposed tight price regulations on medicines and procedures to control health care costs for individuals and ensure access to basic care. These price caps,

Figure 2.1
The Change in Structure of China's National Health Expenditures

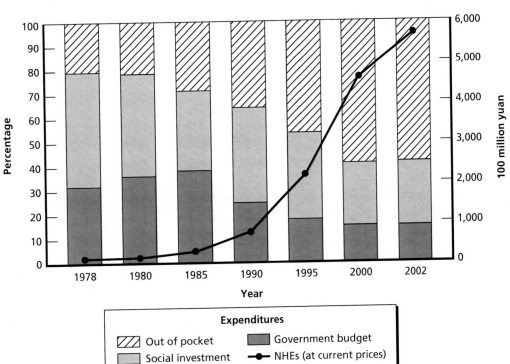

SOURCE: Data from Project Team of the Development Research Center of the State Council of China (2005), Chapter Two, Tables 1 and 3.
RAND OP212-2.1

however, had numerous unintended consequences. Problems included the emergence of a black market (where patients were charged a fee that exceeded the regulated price), overprovision of profitable high-tech services, and overuse of prescription drugs (Liu and Lu, 2000; Eggleston and Yip, 2004). An estimated 52 percent of China's health care spending now goes to drugs, compared with the worldwide average of 15 percent (World Bank, 2004; Meng et al., 2005). Consequently, despite price regulations, health care costs have been increasing considerably and are skewed toward outpatient and prescription drug costs.

There were also dramatic changes in the rural health care system. After 1982 the rural economic system changed from the collective economy under the communes to one based on individual household decisions. As a result of this change, the CMS collapsed rapidly as it lost its institutional base for fund-raising (Project Team of the Development Research Center of the State Council of China, 2005). According to a national rural health service survey in 1985, only 5 percent of administrative villages still implemented the CMS, compared with 90 percent in the past (Cai, 1998). Without the CMS, Chinese peasants had no way to pool risks for health care expenses, and 900 million rural dwellers, mostly poor citizens, became effectively uninsured. In the meantime, the barefoot doctors became unemployed and were forced to become private health care practitioners. They began working without regulations or continuous training, and their interest shifted from providing a public service to making a profit (Blumenthal and Hsiao, 2005). Drug prices and sales soon exploded in rural areas because former barefoot doctors and clinics found that selling drugs was an easy way of generating profit (Bloom and Gu, 1997).

A survey of 190,000 urban and rural residents conducted by China's Health Ministry in late 2003 found that 36 percent of patients in cities and 39 percent in the countryside avoided seeing doctors because they were unable to afford medical treatment. According to Chinese government figures, hospital visits dropped almost 5 percent between 2000 and 2003, while hospital profits increased 70 percent over the same period (Yu, 2006; Markus, 2004; and Lim, 2006). In the meantime, although the overall incidence of contagious disease in China has continued to drop, some contagious diseases—such as hepatitis, pulmonary tuberculosis, and snail fever (schistosomiasis)—have revived; some endemic diseases, such as HIV, have been expanding in some areas, especially in the economically deprived rural areas (Project Team of the Development Research Center of the State Council of China, 2005).

Recognizing these unintended consequences and public discontent, China's leaders are considering yet another round of health care reform. The government has proposed a social medical-insurance system that would include both urban and rural insurance components.[2] To date, no official plans have been announced.

Health System Evolution in India

India's current health policy originated in the nation-building activities that occurred during independence in 1947 and in the philosophy embodied in the government of India's 1946 *Report on the Health Survey and Development Committee*, commonly referred to as the *Bhore Committee Report* (Gupte, Ramachandran, and Mutatkar, 2001; Peters et al., 2002). The report concluded that India's poor health conditions could be attributed to unsanitary conditions,

---

[2]   Individual health savings accounts are an example of an urban component.

defective nutrition, the inadequacy of the existing medical and preventive health organization, and a lack of health education. The committee provided comprehensive recommendations that included placing health workers on the public payroll and limiting the need for private practitioners. It also emphasized preventive methods and the threat of communicable diseases. Moreover, the recommendations included an infrastructure plan for a three-tier health care system at the district level to provide preventive and curative health care to dwellers in both rural and urban areas. Although many of these recommendations were not implemented at the time, the report helped trigger the reforms that followed (Gupte, Ramachandran, and Mutatkar, 2001). Indian policymakers have made a conscious effort to invest in health services since 1949.

The Bhore Committee laid down the principle that access to primary care is a basic right and should be independent of individual socioeconomic conditions. Consequently, primary health care was established as the foundation of the national health care system. Like China, India's central government acknowledged people's right to access care and the importance of prioritized public health care service. However, India's government never intended to eliminate the private provision of health care. The public-sector focus arose in part because the private sector's involvement with Western medicine was very small at the time of independence (Peters et al., 2002). A three-tiered system similar to China's was developed to, in theory, provide health care to all rural inhabitants. At the lowest level, primary health centers (PHCs) were designed to provide basic medical care, disease prevention, and health education. The next tier, subcenters (SCs), were intended to provide public health services. A top tier of community centers and district hospitals offered specialist services. By the end of the 1980s, an extensive health service infrastructure was developed and substantial numbers of health care personnel were trained: Between 1980 and 1990, the number of PHCs more than tripled from about 5,500 to 20,536 and the number of doctors increased by more than 100,000 (Qadeer, 2000).

Constitutionally, health care delivery in India is largely the responsibility of the provincial states. The central government is in charge of defining policies and providing a national strategic framework, financial resources, and medical education (Qadeer, 2000). Influenced by both the Bhore Committee Report and the *Alma Ata Declaration of Health for All by the Year 2000* (WHO and the United Nation's Children's Fund, 1978), the National Health Policy of 1983 buttressed the rhetoric about establishing a strong national public health services system based on the foundation of decentralized primary health care services. In practice, however, states struggled to maintain and administer health care facilities, and over time they became dependent on the central government for financial and programmatic assistance to implement disease control (Peters, Rao, and Fryatt, 2003). For example, although states now account for 75 to 90 percent of public spending on health, most of these funds go to salaries and wages, making states dependent on the central government's fund for nonwage items such as drugs and equipment (Selvaraju, 2000). Like China, India uses a five-year planning process to determine national goals and priorities. This process reinforces state dependence on the central government and institutionalizes a top-down decisionmaking process that sets priorities; implements centrally sponsored, vertical disease-control programs; and creates plans for health care personnel and facilities (World Bank, 1997; Peters, Rao, and Fryatt, 2003).

Since the 1980s, multiple forces have driven changes in the health system in India. As Qadeer (2000) argues, the emerging middle class and private practitioners worked with international donors to push privatization in the health care system. The middle class lobbied for "high-tech hospitals" that provide international standards of health care; the private practitioners benefited from government subsidies for medical education and put pressure on the authorities to loosen regulations over medical care. International donors, such as the International Monetary Fund and the World Bank, played a crucial role in supporting reforms, including cutting health sector investments, encouraging the private sector, and introducing user fees and private investments in public hospitals. As a result, PHCs suffered a setback in the 1990s. Declining funds for infectious disease–control programs led to a reduction in the services provided by the PHCs and a shift in focus to family planning (Qadeer, 2000). This effect is shown in Figure 2.2, which highlights the changes in health and related investments from the 1950s to the 1990s. There was an increase in the total direct investment in health as well as related investments in water supply and sanitation. The specific investment in family planning rose from less than 1 percent to 26 percent of the total. At the same time, spending on the control of communicable diseases dropped from 17 to 4 percent. Although several communicable diseases such as smallpox and dracunculiasis (Guinea worm disease) were eradicated in the 1970s and 1990s, respectively, vaccine-preventable diseases continued to constitute an estimated 7 percent of disability adjusted life years (DALY) losses nationwide. New diseases such as HIV/AIDS have spread aggressively, and several infectious diseases once considered controlled, such as tuberculosis and malaria, have reemerged as greater public health concerns (Gupte, Ramachandran, and Mutatkar, 2001).

Figure 2.2
Financial Allocations for Health Sectors in India Between 1951 and 1997

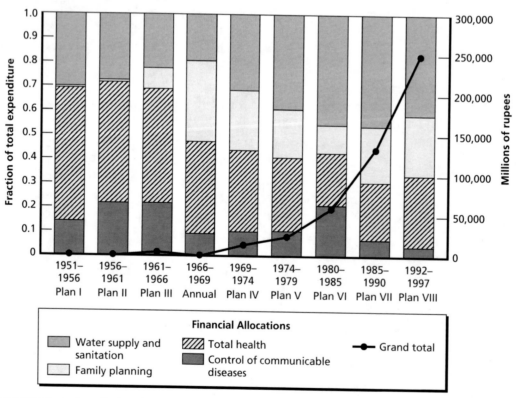

SOURCE: Data from Qadeer (2000), Table 2.
RAND OP212-2.2

Conclusions

An overview of the evolution of the health systems in China and India reveals some similar patterns and striking differences. We summarize the countries' important historical developments and milestones in Table 2.1. Although China and India face very different demographic and health challenges, both countries have achieved great health gains since the late 1940s. However, they have also experienced growing disparities across social classes and geographic areas as well as increasing demands for customized health care. Combined with private business interests, this demand is driving focus away from public health toward individual medical care, and from preventive treatment toward curative treatment. Meanwhile, reduced attention to and investment in public health, especially the prevention of communicable diseases, has resulted in the reemergence of some diseases and expanded health inequalities.

This retrospective review aims to provide readers with a better understanding of how the health systems of China and India have evolved and reached their current forms. In the next three chapters, we discuss and compare the current systems of the two countries along dimensions of current overall performance, intermediate outcomes, and policy levers.

Table 2.1
History of Health Systems in China and India

Period	Indicators	China	India
Late 1940s to early 1980s	Strategies or policies	Priority given to preventive care and health education	Priority given to curative care
	Providers or entities	Completely publicly owned; CMS delivers care in rural areas; a three-tiered system is established	Public and private providers coexist; a three-tiered system is established
	Health gains	Substantial	Moderate
Early 1980s to early 2000s	Disease trend	Chronic diseases replace infectious diseases as top causes of death; aging population	Infectious disease remains the top cause of death; HIV/AIDS spreads aggressively
	Providers or entities	CMS collapses; emerging privatization	Further privatization; PHCs suffer a setback
Early 2000s to present	Policy context	Health system reform	No clear action taken

CHAPTER THREE

Overall Performance in Achieving Ultimate Ends

The WHO's 2000 report entitled *The World Health Report 2000—Health Systems: Improving Performance* states that a health system should have three fundamental objectives:

- improving the health of the population it serves
- responding to people's expectations
- providing financial protection against the costs of ill health.

In this chapter, we compare how China and India fare in achieving these goals.

Health Status

Key Health Indicators
Overall, people in China live longer and are healthier than people in India (see Table 3.1). According to WHO's statistics, a woman born in India in 2004 has a life expectancy of 63 years, whereas a woman born in China at the same time has a life expectancy of 74 years. A man born in India has a life expectancy of 61 years, whereas a man born in China has a life expectancy of 70 years. The disparity in life expectancy between the two countries is greater for women than for men, which is partly a result of the ten-fold greater maternal death rate during childbirth for women in India compared with women in China. Additionally, residents of India suffer higher mortality rates in both childhood and adulthood than do residents of China.

Table 3.1
Key Health Indicators

Country	Life Expectancy in Years, 2004			Probability of Death, 2004[a]						Maternal Death Rate, 2000[b]	LBW Rate, 1999[c]
				≤1 Year	< 5 Years			15 to 60 Years			
	M or F	M	F	M or F	M or F	M	F	M	F		
China	72	70	74	27	31	27	36	158	99	56	6
India	62	61	63	58	85	81	89	275	202	540	30

NOTES: M = male; F = female.

[a] Per 1,000 persons.

[b] Per 100,000 women.

[c] Per 100 newborns.

Health status at birth in India is poor. In 2004 it was estimated that 30 percent of infants in India were born with low birth weight (LBW, less than 2,500 grams at birth), whereas only 6 percent of newborns in China were born with LBW. Fifty-eight out of every 1,000 infants in India died before their first birthday, whereas only 27 out of every 1,000 infants in China died before their first birthday.[1]

Other Vital Health Indicators

In addition to life expectancy and mortality rates, significant differences exist between the two countries in other important health indicators. For example, India has many more deaths due to communicable diseases. Table 3.2 summarizes death rates, categorized by cause, in both countries in 2000. In China, noncommunicable diseases accounted for 77 percent of all deaths. Heart disease, chronic obstructive pulmonary disease, and cancer accounted for approximately 67 percent of all deaths. Among infectious diseases, only lower respiratory infections, hepatitis B virus infection and tuberculosis, and perinatal conditions contributed to relatively significant mortality. In India, on the other hand, communicable and noncommunicable diseases each caused more than 40 percent of all deaths. Compared with China, India had much higher

Table 3.2
Death Rates by Cause

Cause of Death	Deaths (per 100,000 persons)	
	China	India
All causes	701.5	988.8
Lower uncertainty bound	669.0	950.8
Upper uncertainty bound	731.7	1,017.4
Communicable, maternal, perinatal, and nutritional conditions	83.7	401.9
Infectious and parasitic diseases	39.0	197.3
Tuberculosis	20.8	34.8
Sexually transmitted diseases, excluding HIV	0.0	4.6
HIV/AIDS	3.3	34.4
Diarrheal diseases	8.3	43.5
Childhood-cluster diseases	1.6	27.4
Meningitis	0.6	5.1
Hepatitis B	1.5	2.2
Hepatitis C	0.6	0.9
Malaria	0.0	0.9

---

[1] Note that unlike the rest of the world, where child mortality is higher in males than in females, female child mortality exceeded male child mortality in both China and India according to a 2004 estimate. In China, girls had a 33 percent higher risk of dying than their male counterparts during the first five years of life. These inequities are thought to "arise from the preferential treatment of boys in family health care-seeking behavior and in nutrition" (WHO, 2006).

Table 3.2—Continued

Cause of Death	Deaths (per 100,000 persons)	
	China	India
Respiratory infections	22.4	107.0
Maternal conditions	0.8	12.7
Perinatal conditions	20.9	72.6
Nutritional deficiencies	0.6	12.3
Noncommunicable diseases	541.4	486.9
Malignant neoplasms	133.5	71.0
Other neoplasms	1.2	1.2
Diabetes mellitus	9.6	14.9
Endocrine disorders	2.4	1.5
Neuropsychiatric conditions	8.0	17.4
Sense organ diseases	NA	0.1
Cardiovascular diseases	230.5	267.7
Respiratory diseases	110.0	58.1
Digestive diseases	27.9	32.6
Genitourinary diseases	10.7	11.2
Skin diseases	NA	0.7
Musculoskeletal diseases	1.0	0.7
Congenital anomalies	6.6	9.9
Oral conditions	NA	0.0
Injuries	76.3	100.0
Unintentional injuries	52.3	76.2
Intentional injuries	24.0	23.8

NOTE: NA = not available.

SOURCE: WHO, 2004.

death rates due to HIV/AIDS, diarrheal diseases, respiratory infections, and perinatal conditions, but lower rates of cancer and respiratory diseases (WHO, 2004).

As for the prevalence of specific diseases, the epidemic of HIV/AIDS in Asia is expanding rapidly. In 2003, 650,000 Chinese were estimated to be living with HIV. India had the largest number of people living with HIV outside South Africa—5.7 million in 2005. In 2000, there were an estimated 1,856,000 new tuberculosis cases in India and 1,365,000 new cases in China. Approximately 650,000 malaria cases were reported in India in 2004, which represents a 45 percent reduction since 1997. Only 75,000 cases of malaria were found in China in 2003. Obesity and the condition of being overweight are fast-growing problems in both countries.

According to China's 2002 national survey, 7.1 percent of Chinese adults were obese and 22.8 percent were overweight. In India, the obesity rate was 1 percent for males and 4 percent for females in the slums; the corresponding figures among the middle class were 32.3 and 50 percent, respectively (Gupte, Ramachandran, and Mutatkar, 2001). Diabetes is prevalent in both countries, but particularly in India: By 2000, 3 percent of India's population had diabetes, a rate higher than the estimated worldwide prevalence of 2.8 percent (Wild et al., 2004). The number of diabetics in India is projected to reach about 80 million by 2030. In China in 2000 there were approximately 21 million diabetics; this number is expected to double by 2030 (Gupte, Ramachandran, and Mutatkar, 2001). The total number of diabetics in both countries already exceeds that in the United States (Wild et al., 2004).

In summary, India's health status is worse than China's. The disparity is largely the result of causes—such as communicable diseases—that can be addressed by effective health policy.

Financial Risk Protection

Poor health is associated with worse physical and mental well-being. Extensive research has shown that poor health can also increase poverty and reduce material well-being through a number of paths, including excessive medical expense, impaired labor market participation, and loss of productivity (Liu, Rao, and Hsiao, 2003). WHO argues that one of the most important goals of health systems is to distribute and reduce risks throughout society (WHO, 2000).

Unfortunately, the health systems in China and India provide little protection from financial risk. In China, medical expenses have become an important cause of transient (as opposed to chronic) poverty.[2] These expenses have raised the number of rural households living below the poverty line by 44 percent (Liu, Rao, and Hsiao, 2003; Liu and Rao, 2006). A study of 30 randomly selected counties in poor areas in China showed that 25 percent of the surveyed households had to borrow money and that another 6 percent had to sell their assets to pay for health care (Hsiao and Liu, 1996). Because of this high spending, many other household expenditures—e.g., food, tuition, and farming expenses—were crowded out (Wang, Zhang, and Hsiao, 2006).

Similar evidence is observed in India. In 2004 poor Indians spent 40 percent of their income on health care; the rich spent about 2.4 percent (Varatharajan, Thankappan, and Sabeena, 2004). Studies found that medical expenses were one of the three main factors pushing people into poverty (Krishna, 2004). Seventeen to 34 percent of hospitalized patients were impoverished because of medical costs (Peters et al., 2002).

The heavy burden of health costs in China and India is not a surprise, given the lack of well-developed health-insurance schemes in both countries. This high burden is exacerbated by several factors. First, the lack of access to affordable care means that people defer preventive and other necessary care. Consequently, when they do seek care, they typically have a more serious and costly medical condition. Second, for those who seek treatment, physician-induced overutilization of care further increases the financial burden of care.

---

[2] The transient poor are those who move in and out of poverty.

Consumer Satisfaction

WHO's 2000 report also argues that one of the fundamental goals of health systems is to respond to consumer expectations:

> In particular, people have a right to expect that the health system will treat them with individual dignity . . . their needs should be promptly attended to, without long delays in waiting for diagnosis and treatment—not only for better health outcomes but also to respect the value of people's time and to reduce their anxiety. Patients also often expect confidentiality, and to be involved in choices about their own health, including where and from whom they receive care.

Despite its importance, consumer satisfaction has not been widely studied in China or India. A 2001 survey of Chinese patients from three provinces that were selected to represent different stages of economic development revealed that widespread dissatisfaction with public providers, mainly because of high user fees and poor staff attitudes, was driving patients to seek cheaper but lower-quality care from poorly regulated providers (Lim, Yang, Zhang, Feng, et al., 2004). In another survey of patients from ten hospitals in a populous province, patients expressed satisfaction with the hospitals' environment but explicit dissatisfaction with the hospitals' ability to build relationships with patients and keep them informed (Liu and Lu, 2000).

A 1999 patient satisfaction survey in 25 public hospitals in Andhra Pradesh in India found that top patient concerns included corruption among hospital staff, lack of utilities such as water supply and fans, poor maintenance of toilets and general lack of cleanliness, and poor communication and interpersonal skills (Mahapatra, Srilatha, and Sridhar, 2001).

The paucity of data on patient satisfaction in China and India implies that both countries should consider patient satisfaction an important measure of quality of care, but that they do not yet do so.

CHAPTER FOUR

Intermediate Outcomes: Access, Quality, and Efficiency

In Chapter Three, we discussed the current overall performance of the Chinese and Indian health systems vis-à-vis achieving ultimate ends. In this chapter, we discuss the intermediate outcomes (i.e., access, quality, and efficiency) that lead to the overall performance of health systems. Although intermediate outcomes can affect the ultimate ends of a health system, they are "only intermediate and partial results" (Hsiao, 2003).

Access

Access, here defined as *effective availability*, measures how easy it is for people to overcome barriers (e.g., physical, financial, timing, and service availability obstacles) to get care (Roberts et al., 2004). Although both China and India determined that receiving basic health care is a fundamental right, there has been a decline in access to basic care in both countries in the past decade.

Access to care in China has deteriorated. As the focus of care has shifted from preventive to curative care, many public health services (such as immunization and other services to prevent contagious diseases) are no longer available for free. According to a survey conducted by the Chinese Ministry of Health, 80 percent of the public health services were performed at a lower rate than the target set by the ministry, and one-third of the services were provided at less than half the target rate (Project Team of the Development Research Center of the State Council of China, 2005).

There is also evidence of widening inequalities in health care in China. In particular, empirical evidence suggests widening gaps in both financial and physical access to care between rural and urban residents. A survey conducted in 1994 revealed that residents of big cities had better access to health insurance and better access to health facilities compared with those who lived in rural areas (Shi, 1996). From 1980 to 1989, the number of township clinics decreased by 14 percent, and the number of active primary health care workers declined by 36 percent in rural areas (Liu, 2004). In contrast, the number of large hospitals located in cities increased by 56 percent, from 9,478 in 1980 to 14,771 in 1995. Meanwhile, the number of health professionals concentrated in urban facilities increased by 235 percent between 1980 and 1989 (Chinese Ministry of Health, 1994; Chinese Ministry of Health, 1995; and Liu, Hsiao, and Eggleston, 1999). In addition, according to a 1993 national survey, 59 percent of rural patients refused to be hospitalized because of the inability to pay. The comparable proportion was 40 percent among urban dwellers (Chinese Ministry of Health, 1994; Liu, Hsiao, and Eggleston, 1999). As for physical access to care, from 1989 to 1997, distance to the closest clinic decreased by a small amount (about 0.5 km) on average, with the largest decreases occurring in the poorer villages (Akin, Dow, and Lance, 2005).

India too faces access-to-care challenges. In 2005 there were substantial shortfalls at each level of health facility: There were 10 percent fewer SCs and PHCs than needed and 50 percent fewer community health centers (CHCs) than needed (Datar, Mukherji, and Sood, 2007). Transportation may be a serious barrier, since public transportation between PHCs or CHCs and state hospitals is irregular and infrequent, while private transportation is expensive (Ramani and Dileep, 2005). Although access to care is unequal in rural and urban areas in India, that gap appears to be smaller than the one that exists in China. In the case of child immunization in India, for example, the gap between the proportion of rural compared with urban children who received at least one vaccine has narrowed, falling from 18 to 12 percent. However, the proportion of children living in villages with no health facility increased from 43 to 47 percent (Datar, Mukherji, and Sood, 2007). Because almost 80 percent of health care expenses are paid out of pocket by patients, financial barriers constrain both rural residents and the urban poor from seeking care (Ramani and Dileep, 2005).

In summary, both China and India have poor access to care. Consumers bear a disproportionately large burden of health care costs and often lack access to care because of an inability to pay. There is some evidence of rising inequalities in access to care in both countries, but more so in China. Both countries have set ambitious targets for the delivery of essential public health services, including immunizations, but have not yet met these targets.

Quality

Routine evaluation and assessment of quality is an important part of a health system. However, China and India lack national or regional structures charged with conducting routine quality assessments. In China, even when there is an assessment, data are sometimes proven unreliable (Koplan, Xingzhu, and Haichao, 2005).

Both countries are plagued by (1) underuse of key public health services and (2) supply-induced overutilization of new technologies. Extensive research has shown evidence of overuse of high-cost technologies and expensive medications in China, especially antibacterial drugs. Such overuse not only increases the cost of care but might also adversely affect patient health. For example, Meng et al. (2005) examined hospital records and found a trend toward prescribing newly marketed drugs with higher prices; only 13 percent of the money spent on the 15 most often-used drugs was expended on drugs that were considered safe and effective. Liu and Mills (2005) examined detailed records of appendicitis and pneumonia patients and found that more than one-third of drug expenditures were unnecessary. A study that investigated the use of antibiotics in a Chinese hospital in 2000 found that as many as 80 percent of the inpatients used antibiotics, a percentage that far exceeds the international average level (Project Team of the Development Research Center of the State Council of China, 2005).

Overprescription and unnecessary interventions are observed in India as well. For example, 52 percent of out-of-pocket health expenditures paid for medicines and fees, as did 71 percent of inpatient expenditures (Whitehead, Dahlgren, and Evans, 2001); the worldwide average is just 15 percent (World Bank, 2004; Meng et al., 2005). Moreover, care provided by the public sector is repeatedly described as *poor*, and care provided by the private sector, often deemed uneven, has elicited calls for greater regulation (Bhatia and Cleland, 2004; Mills et al.,

2002). An analysis of health care received by female outpatients found that private providers supplied better care in terms of thoroughness of diagnosis and superior doctor-patient communication, but that private providers overprescribed drugs (Bhatia and Cleland, 2004).

In summary, evidence shows that supply-induced overuse of medicines and procedures is a serious problem and that systematic health care quality assessments and controls need to be incorporated into the health care systems of both countries.

Efficiency

The efficiency of a health system is determined by the degree to which the system maximizes the health-status gain of the general population at a minimum cost. There are two kinds of efficiency: *Technical efficiency* means producing outputs in the "right way" at the minimum cost; *allocative efficiency* means producing the "right outputs" to maximize the collective gains (Roberts et al., 2004).

In practice, however, the efficiency of a health system is hard to measure, and proof of efficiency in China and India is rare. The limited evidence that is available suggests that both countries experience technical inefficiency due to the fragmentation and bureaucracy of the national agencies, as discussed in Chapter Three. One specific example in China is the development of multiple agencies equivalent to the U.S. Centers for Disease Control and Prevention (CDC). Aiming to improve disease surveillance, all levels of government founded their own separate CDC equivalents in the late 1990s. However, these CDCs are guided by no well-defined roles, and there are no clear policies that establish how these CDCs should relate to each other. As a result, some local and provincial CDCs have attempted to establish their own "national" capacity (Koplan, Xingzhu, and Haichao, 2005). A specific example in India is the disconnection between horizontal health services (i.e., regular health services) and vertical control programs (i.e., specific disease control programs such as polio eradication). Researchers argue that although vertical control programs can be helpful because they reduce a specific disease burden in the short term, they often lead to disruptions in routine primary health care provision (Devadasan, Boelaert, et al., 2007). Unfortunately, the paucity of evidence does not allow us to draw conclusions regarding the efficiency of the Chinese and Indian health systems.

CHAPTER FIVE

Policy Levers of Health Systems in China and India

As discussed in Chapter One, we adopt an analytical framework that separates a health system into policy levers, intermediate outcomes, and ultimate ends. We compared the overall and intermediate performance of the health systems in China and India in Chapters Three and Four; in this chapter, we discuss in depth how policy levers used in these two countries lead to the current performance of the national health systems.

The following five factors influence the ultimate performance of a health system and can be affected by policy: the financing, payment, and organization of health care delivery; regulation; and consumer behavior.

Financing

Financing refers to the mechanisms by which resources are mobilized to fund health sector activities.[1] Financing has the most important and direct impact on the performance of a health system (Roberts et al., 2004). Except for external aid and donations, which constitute about 1.6 percent of 2003 total health expenditures in India and 0.1 percent of 2003 total health expenditures in China (WHO, 2006), all the money raised domestically through any kind of direct or indirect financing mechanism comes from citizens of the country.

Overall Spending

Health care is normally financed through the following methods: general revenue, social insurance, private insurance, community financing, and out-of-pocket payments. Recent research also suggests that informal payment (in cash or in kind) is an important but often overlooked source of health care finance in developing countries (Lewis, 2007). Although most countries use mixed financing methods for health care, the primary financing method a country chooses determines (1) the amount of money available for health care, (2) who controls the resources, and (3) who bears the financial burden (Hsiao, 2003).

India spent 4.8 percent of its gross domestic product (GDP) on health care in 2003, somewhat less than China's 5.6 percent. Translated into per capita total expenditures at an average exchange rate, however, the Chinese spent an average of $61 compared with India's $27. As Figure 5.1 depicts, China has steadily increased its per capita total spending on health between 1999 and 2003, while India's spending has remained stable.

---

1   Once the money is raised, how it is disbursed or allocated becomes a matter of payment.

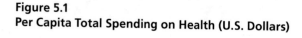

Figure 5.1
Per Capita Total Spending on Health (U.S. Dollars)

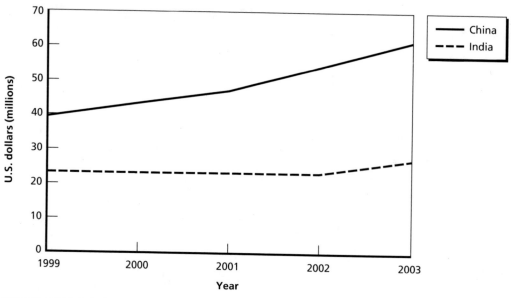

SOURCE: WHO (2006).
RAND OP212-5.1

Compared with other developing countries, China and India spent less of their GDP on health in 2003: Mexico spent 6.2 percent, Brazil and Colombia spent 7.6 percent, and the Czech Republic spent 7.5 percent. Of course, China and India spent very little on health care compared with nations with developed economies. For example, per capita spending in the United States ($5,711) far exceeds spending in China and India. However, it is difficult to determine how much a country *should* spend on health care, and using other countries as benchmarks is not very informative (Savedoff, 2007). For example, similar health spending does not necessarily produce the same health status in different countries; factors such as the epidemiological profile and the effectiveness of health inputs can be substantially different across countries (Savedoff, 2007). In addition, the official GDP and health spending statistics might not be a very reliable measure of true income and spending, since developing country economies tend to have large shadow economies (i.e., unrecorded legal income and proceeds from illicit activities). For example, Schneider and Enste (2002) estimated that the shadow economy of Mexico totaled more than 50 percent of the country's official GDP, while the shadow economy in high-income countries such as Japan totaled less than 10 percent of the official GDP (Schneider and Enste, 2002; Roberts et al., 2004).

Financing Structures

It is therefore more meaningful to scrutinize the structure of health system financing, an area in which China and India share great similarities. As Figure 5.2 shows, the proportion of total medical spending paid out of pocket in 2003 was very high in both countries—56 percent in China and 73 percent in India. General government expenditure constituted the second-largest financing source at 36 percent in China and 25 percent in India. The remaining financing sources—prepaid plans, other private funds, and external aid—constituted less than 8 percent of total health spending in China and about 2 percent in India. The high proportion of

Figure 5.2
Health Care Financing Structures in China and India in 2005

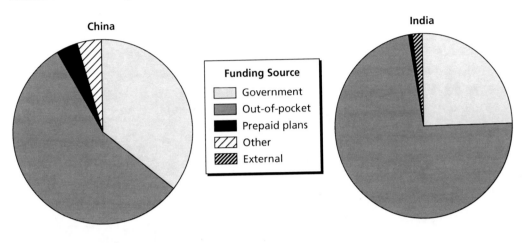

SOURCE: WHO (2006).
RAND *OP212-5.2*

care financed by out-of-pocket payment is quite common in most developing countries, where it ranges from 50 to 60 percent; 2004 rates in the United States (13 percent) and United Kingdom (10 percent) were much lower (Pauly et al., 2006). However, it is worth noting that a low rate of out-of-pocket payments is not confined only to residents of rich countries. Some developing countries have achieved rather low rates as well: In 2003 in Mozambique the percentage was 15, and in Thailand it was 29 (WHO, 2006). In addition, high out-of-pocket payments in developing countries are not concentrated among only the most affluent consumers; rather, the distribution of such payments spreads across the whole income scale; therefore, out-of-pocket payments potentially consume a large share of family income (Wagstaff, Watanabe, and van Doorslaer, 2001; Pauly et al., 2006).

A less apparent but common source of health care financing in developing countries is informal payments (called "red packages"[2] in China and "under-the-table payments" elsewhere). These in-kind or cash payments are made by patients to providers "outside official payment channels" and are meant to cover purchases that should be paid for by the health care system (Lewis, 2007). These payments help patients receive better (or any) care or jump the queue. Informal payment is common in both China and India. According to a variety of data sources, it is estimated that 26 percent of residents of India made informal payments for health care between 1992 and 2002. More than 70 percent of Chinese hospital patients gave providers red packages, and outpatients paid average red packages of 140 to 320 yuan ($16 to $36) per hospital visit (Lewis, 2007; Ensor, 2004; and Bloom, Han, and Li, 2000). Additionally, providers and hospitals often receive pharmaceutical company kickbacks in the form of cash, cars, mobile phones, entertainment, and travel. Although there is little information about the extent of kickbacks, it is estimated that a midsize hospital's kickback "earnings" could match the typical government grant (Bloom, Han, and Li, 2000). Unsurprisingly, informal payments go largely unreported, and it is unclear to what extent the officially reported out-of-pocket payments include such informal payments.

---

2   Red packages are named after the traditional red wrapping that covers gifts or payments of cash in China.

The Role of Insurance

Unlike other consumption expenses, medical spending is largely unpredictable both in timing and quantity, and therefore risks can be very high. A key drawback of out-of-pocket payments is that they do not pool risks; this places a greater financial burden on poor and sick people and often bankrupts patients and their families. Risk pooling, however, effectively insures people against such risks by transferring the costs of covering the sick to a large number of healthy people who need only pay a small amount (i.e., a premium). Risk pooling assumes that a large number of people with different levels of risk participate in the process and that the loss-producing events are not highly correlated (Pauly et al., 2006).

In recent years, policymakers in China and India have focused on the potential to use private or social health insurance as a way to pool risk. Both countries used to rely mainly on heavily subsidized public providers that the national health service implicitly insured. Like many other developing countries, however, China and India have sought to replace the old system with formal public or private insurance schemes and to separate purchasers (i.e., insurers) from providers to introduce more competition and thereby curtail costs.

Public health insurance has played an important role in China over the past decade. In 1998, the State Council established a public insurance program, aiming to replace formerly heavily subsidized public health care services with a formal social insurance scheme. That scheme, comprising a medical savings account (MSA) and a social risk pool fund, provides a basic benefit package to all urban workers, including employees of public and private enterprises. The insurance covers costs of basic outpatient and inpatient health services as well as catastrophic expenses up to a set limit (The Central Party Committee and the State Council of China, 1997; The State Council of China, 1998). Under this new scheme, employees contribute 2 percent of their pay and employers contribute 6 percent of their employee payroll. By the end of 2003, the MSA covered 109 million people, less than a quarter of the total workforce. The social risk pool fund was less than 1 percent of the GDP in 2003 (Chinese Ministry of Labor and Social Security, 2004). This new scheme, however, does not cover workers' dependents, the unemployed, or most of the self-employed. As a result, the proportion of urban residents without health insurance rose from 27 to 50 percent between 1993 and 2003. On the other hand, private insurance is still scarce (Drechsler and Jütting, 2005; Chinese Ministry of Health, n.d. [2003]).

Moreover, nearly 80 percent of residents in rural areas had no insurance at all by 2003, because of the collapse of the CMS (Chinese Ministry of Health, n.d. [2003]). The Chinese government recently announced the reestablishment of some forms of community-based health insurance, whose features include voluntary enrollment, basic and catastrophic coverage, and low premiums (but high copayments). However, studies have found that even small premiums discourage enrollment and high copayments deter poor participants from seeking care; therefore, the richer farmers benefit more from such insurance (Wang et al., 2005).

According to an Organisation for Economic Co-operation and Development (OECD) report, Hong Kong and India are the only middle-income Asian countries or regions that do not have obligatory public health insurance (Drechsler and Jütting, 2005). In 1999 India's parliament passed the Insurance Regulatory and Development Authority Bill, which allows private-sector entities to enter the health services market by providing health insurance, and which envisages the creation of a regulatory authority that would oversee operations in the insurance market (Mahal, 2002). Despite projections that India has great market potential for private health insurance (Sekhri and Savedoff, 2005; Drechsler and Jütting, 2005), private insurance still constitutes a small fraction of total financing sources: Approximately 1 percent of total health expenditures in India, and approximately just 3 percent of the population, was covered by private prepayment plans in 2003 (WHO, 2006; Devadasan, Ranson, et al., 2006).

Although India still does not have a clear agenda for developing public or social insurance, the National Rural Health Mission proposed supporting community-based health insurance schemes (CHIs) by subsidizing premiums for the poor (Mathur, 2005). Some nongovernmental organizations have initiated a variety of CHI experiments that aim to ease the burden on the poor, but most of these experiments depend on external resources for financial sustainability (Devadasan et al., 2006). Two studies assessed willingness to pay for health insurance among rural and poor residents in India. Dror, Radermacher, and Koren (2007) reported that 30 percent of poor people are willing to spend up to 2 percent of their annual household income on a health insurance premium. In a different study, Dror et al. (2007) found that among the poor, generally illiterate respondents, 73 percent would like to choose some type of insurance package and only 27 percent would decide to pay nothing. These positive findings shed some light on the potential of CHIs as a policy option to finance health care.

In summary, both China and India rely heavily on financing health care via out-of-pocket payments. Both countries face the challenge of reducing the burden and risk of health care costs. The policy focus in China is to rely on social or public insurance mechanisms to reduce this burden. In contrast, India is betting on the emergence of private micro–health insurance policies to reduce financial risks associated with health care among the poor. It remains to be seen which policies each country will adopt and whether they will be successful.

Payment

Payment describes how the money, once raised, is spent: who to pay, what to pay for, and how much to pay. Payment is an essential component of any health system because "these [payment] decisions create powerful incentives that influence the actions of all the organizations and individuals in the health care system" (Roberts et al., 2004).

The fee-for-service (FFS) payment method dominates in both China and India. Under FFS, health service providers generally are reimbursed a fee for each service provided (such as a doctor visit, injection, or laboratory test); therefore, providers have an incentive to promote an excessive use of services, resulting in an increase in costs (Barnum, Kutzin, and Saxenian, 1995; Yip and Eggleston, 2001).

The most dominant payment method in India is FFS. Although India has set goals to provide inexpensive public health care to the people, only 0.9 percent of the country's GDP is spent on public-sector health programs, and public health facilities are often understaffed and overcrowded (Mullan, 2006). Therefore, most patients, regardless of income level, go to FFS private practitioners and pay out of pocket instead of using the "free" services provided by the public sector (Mahal, 2003). According to a 1999 survey, 70 percent of private providers charged on a FFS basis. Among those who charged fees for services, most providers indicated that medical associations had little influence on price setting, and only 11 percent of the providers based their prices on the association's recommendations (Bhat, 1999). One of the consequences of rampant use of the FFS model is that curative medicine and specialization are more valuable to providers and family medicine as a discipline is "virtually nonexistent" (Mullan, 2006).

Aiming to control cost and guarantee universal access to basic care, China has established a unique FFS payment model whose distorted pricing system allows the government to set prices for services, procedures, and drugs. To be fair, the tension between the providers and payers is natural and common, with providers tending to charge as much as possible and payers wanting to pay as little as possible. Many countries, including the United States, use government-administered price setting to establish health care payments. For example, U.S. Medicare uses a fee schedule that most private insurers use to set their prices. Unlike countries whose mutually acceptable payment level is reached through bilateral negotiation between providers and payers, China's fees are primarily decided by the government and therefore often represent a purposefully underestimated cost. Providers and hospitals cannot charge patients more than the set price and the central and local governments subsidize the revenue shortfall, which can total up to 60 percent of a hospital's operating revenue (Yip and Eggleston, 2004). However, the government has reduced its promised subsidies since the early 1990s and hospitals and providers have been forced to generate more revenue to compensate. They have found a degree of financial salvation in overprescribing high-technology diagnostic procedures and expensive prescription drugs that are not subject to the pricing scheme. As previously noted, providers and hospitals also receive kickbacks from pharmaceutical companies. Consequently, 52 percent of China's total health care spending goes to drugs, compared with 10 to 19 percent in OECD countries (World Bank, 2004; Meng et al., 2005). The incidence of unnecessary care often increases when the financial incentives are strong (Liu and Mills, 2005). Caesarean sections are overused in China, where they occur during 40 to 50 percent of births in some areas (Project Team of the Development Research Center of the State Council of China, 2005). By comparison, Caesarean sections occur in 25 percent of births in the United States and Canada (Anderson, 2004). Historically, the WHO has estimated that Caesarean sections occur in a maximum of 15 percent of births in a normal population. Without solid scientific evidence that Caesarean sections offer advantages over vaginal delivery, the excessively high rate in China is believed to be partly attributable to supply-induced demand driven up by doctors and hospitals who may be misleading patients about the benefits of Caesarian sections (Project Team of the Development Research Center of the State Council of China, 2005).

Several payment reform experiments have been carried out in China. Yip and Eggleston (2004) found that a prepayment scheme implemented in Hainan Province in 1997 was associated with a slower increase in spending on expensive drugs and high-technology services, compared with FFS schemes.

In conclusion, both China and India rely on a FFS payment system to pay health care providers. This system has created incentives for the overuse of health care services and has further increased the burden on consumers. In China, these problems are exacerbated by the government-administered price-setting process that rules out bilateral negotiation between the government and providers. In India, on the contrary, governments or professional associations have little influence on prices. Both countries face the challenge of reforming the payment system to reduce incentives for overuse and to emphasize the use of cost-effective health care technologies. Savings from such reform could be passed on to consumers, consequently reducing their share of health care expenses.

Organization

Organization refers to the broad structure that organizes health care provision, including ownership, market competition, decentralization (i.e., the delegation of responsibilities among different levels of government), and vertical integration (i.e., coordination among preventive, primary, secondary, and tertiary care providers). How care provision is organized and managed affects the efficiency and quality of the service delivered (Hsiao, 2003).

China: Public Entities Dominate

In the past, China relied solely on public health care entities (e.g., providers, hospitals, financing mechanisms) to provide health care. During economic reforms in 1982, private medical practice was once again allowed in China. In 2000 the central government issued the first regulations concerning nonprofit and for-profit health care organizations (Liu et al., 2006). Today, although China's economy as a whole is dominated by the private sector, the private sector's role in health care is still limited. By 2002 there were more than 200,000 private practitioners, representing about 4 percent of the total 5.2 million health professionals in China; most of these private practitioners were located in rural areas. In that same year, approximately 12 percent of the hospitals were private (Liu et al., 2006). In 2006 a U.S. company acquired a formerly state-owned hospital and turned it into a members-only health maintenance organization (HMO) akin to California's Kaiser Permanente (Lee and Yi, 2006). Although many public hospitals are now allowed to contract out their management services (Lipson, 2004), the government approaches the ownership of hospitals with caution because of concerns that for-profit hospitals might reduce access to and the efficiency of health care. Therefore, current Chinese policy does not subsidize private hospitals and does not exempt for-profit hospitals from taxes (Eggleston and Yip, 2004). Under this policy, the health care market in China is in effect controlled by a government-led monopoly: Public hospitals benefit from many policy advantages, such as tax breaks and revenue subsidies, while private hospitals must compete without such benefits. As Eggleston and Yip (2004) project, unless policies otherwise subsidize access through expanded insurance or subsidize providers for serving the poor and uninsured, competition for patients under distorted FFS prices will *reduce* rather than increase access for those who cannot afford to pay for care. This is because providers will intentionally drop unprofitable basic services.

Given that China is a large country that mostly relies on public provision of health care services, the three-tier, bottom-up delivery system was once regarded as highly efficient for decentralizing health care provision. It was also considered reasonably good at providing basic preventive care to most people, especially those in rural areas. However, according to the analysis of the Project Team of the Development Research Center of the State Council of China (2005), the share of China's health investments in big urban hospitals increased substantially between 1990 and 2002, diminishing resources for rural and community clinics. As a result, urban hospitals are crowded, leaving low-end clinics often underused. At the same time, government spending on public health, such as epidemic prevention, decreased from 27 percent in 1990 to less than 20 percent in 2001 (Project Team of the Development Research Center of the State Council of China, 2005).

India: Private Entities Dominate

Although the Indian government has also made efforts to promote its public health services, it has never—unlike China—used political regulations to sweep out private practitioners. On the contrary, because India's public health system is underfunded, the need for health care services has been filled by a large number of heterogeneous, private health care providers that operate on an FFS basis. The private sector now dominates the health system: 77.4 percent of all health expenditures occurred in private health facilities in 2002 (De Costa and Diwan, 2007). Approximately 70 percent of hospitals are private, and 60 to 79 percent of qualified doctors work in the private sector (Bhat, 1996; Ramani and Dileep, 2005; and WHO, 2006). According to De Costa and Diwan (2007), in 2004 in Madhya Pradesh, a large and relatively poor Indian province, 18,757 out of 24,807 qualified doctors (75.6 percent) worked in the private sector, and 80 percent of those doctors worked in urban areas.

On the public side, India has developed a three-tiered system similar to China's. PHCs were designed to provide basic medical care, disease prevention services, and health education. However, since the early 1990s, PHCs have seen funding decline for infectious-disease control programs: Spending on the control of communicable diseases dropped from 20 to 4 percent between 1980 and 1997. Therefore, PHCs have shifted their services to focus largely on family planning (Qadeer, 2000). In light of this trend, researchers argue that vertical health programs such as family planning and polio eradication, although necessary in certain circumstances, have led to disruptions in general health care services (Devadasan, Boelaert, et al., 2007).

Although there are concerns about the quality of private practitioners, direct systematic comparisons of the quality of care offered by public and private sectors are lacking. Another factor that affects the supply of physicians is that medical students increasingly prefer to work in the private sector; in addition, many emigrate to wealthy countries. Almost 60,000 Indian physicians, equal to 10 percent of the total physicians in India, practice in the United States, United Kingdom, Canada, or Australia (Mullan, 2006).

Comparing Organization in China and India

Comparing China's organization of health care with India's reveals some interesting insights. First, in the early years after their independence, both countries emphasized a public health care system that was equitable and provided basic health care services. This public provision of health care was largely successful in China, but less so in India, which struggled to provide basic health services to its citizens. Consequently, from the 1950s to 1980s, China experienced much larger gains in health compared with India. For example, WHO statistics show that average Chinese life expectancy at birth in 2003 was ten years longer than the Indian life expectancy. Why China's public-sector care was so much more effective is not entirely clear. Part of the difference may be related to the greater centralized control exerted in China.

In the 1980s both countries faced pressure to increase the role of the private sector in providing health care services. This time India was more successful than China in achieving a smoother transition. This could be explained by the fact that, in contrast to China, India did not eliminate the private sector in the years after independence. Therefore, this sector matured gradually to meet the increasing demand for private health care services made by citizens who were unhappy with public health care providers. However, the transition to private provision of health care has come at a cost in both countries. Citizens of both countries now bear greater financial burdens and risks in financing their health care needs. There is also now an increased emphasis on individual care and less emphasis on public health. Similarly, the incentives of the private sector are aligned with providing curative rather than preventive treatments. This reduction in attention to public health, especially the prevention of communicable diseases, might be one of the most important emerging issues facing both countries.

Regulation

Regulation refers to the government's use of coercive power to impose a full range of legal constraints (such as laws, administrative rules, and guidelines issued by delegated professional institutes) on organizations and individuals (Roberts et al., 2004).[3] Regulation is fundamental to the success of a health system because "it reduces exposure to disease through enforcement of sanitary code, ensures the timely followup of health hazards, and monitors the quality of medical services and products" (Das Gupta and Rani, 2004).

China: Coercion

As a socialist country, China has a reputation for using coercive political power to closely regulate public services—including health care—through laws, codes, administrative rules, and price setting. However, since the government's restructuring in 1998, the power to regulate and plan for health services has been largely decentralized to the provincial level. At the national level, this power has been divided among several parallel agencies. The Ministry of Health provides general policy guidelines but has modest power to enforce its policies because it does not directly finance health care or enforce regulations. It is the Ministry of Finance that decides the central government's budget for health and government employee insurance. Since family planning is a high priority for the country, the Family Planning Commission has become a powerful agency that controls and manages family planning (Hsiao, 1995). Moreover, after 1998 two new agencies entered the health system. The State General Administration of Quality Supervision, Inspection and Quarantine was established to regulate and monitor port quarantine. The State Food and Drug Administration, split from the Ministry of Health, is responsible for approving health-related products and regulating pricing (Project Team of the Development Research Center of the State Council of China, 2005). As a result of this complex structure, the regulation and enforcement power has been diffused, and policies from different ministries and commissions often conflict with each other. The outbreak of severe acute respiratory syndrome (SARS) in 2003 exposed the structural deficiencies and lack of communication in the public health system (Liu, 2004; Koplan, Xingzhu, and Haichao, 2005). Furthermore, China lacks a system to monitor the quality of health service (Hsiao, 1995).

Finally, even when regulations are successfully implemented, they do not always achieve their goals; sometimes they result in unintended consequences. For example, the price control policies that govern hospitals and drugs have been found ineffective at containing expenditures. Empirical evidence has revealed problems of supply-induced overuse (Liu and Lu, 2000; Meng et al., 2005; Project Team of the Development Research Center of the State Council of China, 2005).

---

3   Please note that according to the definition of *regulation* supplied in Roberts et al. (2004), the constraints that insurers impose on providers are not regarded as regulations because "they are not legal rules imposed by government, but rather contract terms negotiated between buyer and seller."

India: Laissez-Faire

According to India's Constitution, government responsibility for health services is divided into lists—the Union list, the State list, and the Concurrent list—that specify responsibilities for the central government and the state government. The Concurrent list describes responsibilities shared between levels of government, including the prevention of infectious diseases and family planning (Das Gupta and Rani, 2004). In general, though public health is deemed a state subject in India, the policy development and program design are centralized.

At the national level, the Organization of Ministry of Health and Family Welfare consists of the Department of Health, the Department of Family Welfare, and the Department of Indian Systems of Medicine and Homeopathy. This structure has not been regarded as highly effective. In a World Bank survey of senior officials from India's health-related agencies, regulation and enforcement were ranked as the second worst among essential public health functions (Das Gupta and Rani, 2004). Respondents expressed serious concerns about the Organization of Ministry of Health and Family Welfare's capability for monitoring legislation, enforcing laws and regulations, and partnering with state governments.

As for private health providers and insurers, the Indian government—in contrast to China's, which has opted for tight regulation—has adopted a laissez-faire policy. The rapid growth of the private sectors—which has occurred in the absence of any kind of public regulation, mandatory registration, regular service evaluations, quality control, or even self-regulation—has raised many concerns, most of which focus on quality of care (Qadeer, 2000; Ramani and Dileep, 2005). Although a few state or local governments have promulgated regulations for the private health sector, such as the Nursing Home Acts of Delhi and Bombay, most states have no such legislation or are incompletely implementing existing regulations (Bhat, 1996). On the other hand, professional bodies (like the Medical Council of India) that govern the medical profession by providing a code of conduct for practitioners can influence provider behavior. However, a large number of private providers do not belong to professional associations and therefore may not follow association guidelines (Bhat, 1996). As a result, when the Medical Council finds a drug or a technology harmful, it cannot effectively keep doctors from using it; individual doctors have freedom to practice as they choose (Qadeer, 2000). Another concern is physician emigration to wealthy countries: Doctors in India are educated directly (e.g., in public medical schools) or indirectly (e.g., in private medical schools that receive many government benefits) at public expense, yet there is no regulation concerning doctors who depart the country.

In sum, both countries lack a coherent regulatory framework. China's lack of regulatory capability in the public health system has been exacerbated by structural deficiencies and lack of communication between different governmental branches. India's regulation of the private sector is less stringent, and laws are more loosely enforced in both the private and public sectors.

Behavior

In addition to formal regulations, governments and the private sector have another powerful way of achieving health system goals: "influencing people's beliefs, expectations, lifestyles, and preferences through advertising, education, and information dissemination" (Hsiao, 2003). After all, individual behaviors play a salient role in promoting health. Roberts et al. (2004)

argue that four categories of individual behavior should be considered for use as policy levers: treatment-seeking behaviors, health professional behaviors, patient compliance behaviors, and lifestyle and prevention behaviors. Because many of these areas have not been extensively studied, our discussion focuses on changes to lifestyle and prevention behaviors.

During the planned-economy period, the Chinese government frequently launched mass movements and information campaigns to disseminate public health knowledge and promote particular behaviors. In 1952, for example, the State Council formally established Patriotic Health Campaign committees at all administrative levels to enhance awareness of the importance of public health, popularize health knowledge, eliminate insect pests, and improve sanitation (Project Team of the Development Research Center of the State Council of China, 2005). To this day, short and easily remembered slogans are often used as convenient and effective means of disseminating policies and messages to the general population. Giant roadside billboards that promote health campaigns and birth control, such as boards that claim "it is good to have just one child," are ubiquitous, although harsh and insensitive slogans have been recently reexamined and banned.

In recent years, as the prevalence of chronic diseases such as diabetes and hypertension has steadily increased, China has engaged in educational programs to promote healthy behaviors such as smoking cessation, increased physical activity, and increased breast-feeding (Wang et al., 2005; Huang et al., 1994). There have also been campaigns to disseminate information on public health subjects such HIV/AIDS prevention. At the same time, persuasion efforts undertaken by the private sector, including extensive drug advertisements, have caused concerns about potential supply-induced demand for health care and the promotion of unhealthy lifestyles.[4]

India has also recognized the importance of health promotion. At the national level, the Central Health Education Bureau, New Delhi, was established to educate people about health by informing, motivating, and helping them adopt and maintain healthy lifestyles (Das Gupta and Rani, 2004). India's health promotion programs have several strengths, including a well-trained workforce and a school curriculum that incorporates health education (Sharma, 2005).

Compared with China's education system, however, India's has traditionally emphasized advanced education and neglected basic education. As a result, almost 40 percent of the Indian population is illiterate (compared to just 7 percent in China), and therefore the use of print media to convey health messages is controversial (Sharma, 2005). Folk media (i.e., puppets, drama, storytelling, and music) and visual media (i.e., television shows, musicals, and advertisement) are believed to be more effective.

In general, the means and effectiveness of persuasion efforts in both countries have not been well studied, although there is some evidence that health education and promotion campaigns initiated by the Chinese government were effective in the past.

---

4   For instance, although tobacco advertising was banned in China in 1992, tobacco companies circumvent the regulations by sponsoring sports and cultural events.

Summary

To capture the extensive evidence and discussion presented in this chapter, and to highlight the marked differences between the two countries, Table 5.1 displays Chinese and Indian policy levers and indicators.

Table 5.1
Policy Levers Used in the Chinese and Indian Health Systems

Policy Levers	Indicators	China	India
Financing	Total per capita expenditure on health (2003)	$61	$27
	Percentage of national GDP spent on health (2003)	5.6	4.8
	Out-of-pocket expenses as a percentage of total medical spending (2003)	56.0	73.0
	General government contributions as a percentage of total medical spending (2003)	36.0	25.0
	Health insurance composition	Reliance on public insurance	Private microinsurance is emerging
Payment	FFS	Dominant; government sets price	Dominant; providers set price
Organization	Public providers as a percentage of total medical service provision (in China in 2002; in India in 2003)	·96.0	21.0
	Private providers as a percentage of total medical service provision	4.0	79.0
Regulation	Enforcement	Coercive	Laissez-faire
	Regulatory structure	Diffuse	Very diffuse
Behavior	Education and promotion campaigns	Somewhat effective	Limited by illiteracy

SOURCE: WHO (2006).

CHAPTER SIX

Policy Implications

Both China and India have achieved substantial health gains since independence. Nevertheless, each country's health system faces challenges, some common to both countries and some unique. We conclude this paper by identifying key challenges and policy implications and describing the lessons that China and India can learn from each other.

Key Challenges and Associated Policy Implications

Reduce the Out-of-Pocket Burden on Individual Consumers

Both countries rely heavily on out-of-pocket health care payments. However, as many health economists have argued, "moving away from out-of-pocket to prepayment mechanisms is the key to reducing financial catastrophe" (Xu et al., 2007). This challenge can be met by providing the nationalized or social insurance common in Europe, or by encouraging the private insurance common in the United States. India seems to be leaning toward a greater role for private insurance, while China seems to be leaning toward nationalized insurance. We recommend that neither country exclude any sort of insurance; rather, both public and private insurance models and their adapted versions should be considered in each country to meet diverse needs. Both countries should also consider an HMO model that vertically integrates the provision of health insurance and health care to contain costs.

Reduce Overutilization of Services

Reductions in the overutilization of services can be accomplished by moving away from regulated prices and fee-for-service type contracts. Both countries should consider separating drug prescribing and dispensing and should adopt alternative reimbursement mechanisms (such as the prospective payment model adopted by Medicare in the United States). Furthermore, to ensure quality of care, each country must make quality assessment and evaluation an integral part of its health system. Developing and encouraging a culture of professionalism in health care could also help improve quality of care.

Increase Access to Care for the Poor

Although certain health care services are overutilized in China and India because of supply-induced demand, both countries also face the critical problems associated with disadvantaged and underserved populations. China and India need to spend more resources on building primary health care facilities, especially those that provide preventive and basic curative care. They should pay special attention to improving access to care in the rural areas through measures such as education, screening, immunization, and transportation assistance. Finally, existing facilities require more resources and better management.

Build Capacity for Addressing and Monitoring Emerging Diseases (Such as HIV and Obesity)

Both China and India need to improve horizontal and vertical coordination between government branches in the area of communicable disease surveillance and control. China needs to make its data more transparent and reliable; India needs to develop a more effective surveillance system by investing more resources in the system without interrupting routine primary care.

Match Hospital Capabilities with Local Needs

Both countries, but especially China, suffer from an inefficient health care delivery system that is overly concentrated in urban areas and thin in rural and remote areas. Policies that ensure capital and human resources for preventive and basic curative care will help lower-tier clinics and community hospitals continue to exist and improve.

What Can China Learn from India?

Despite statistics that indicate that China has better health outcomes than India and that the Chinese government has committed more resources to health care, China's overall health system performance ranked only 144th out of 191 countries, well behind India's rank of 112th (WHO, 2000). Our comparison of the two countries suggests that China should consider two particular aspects of India's health care system: (1) greater private-sector involvement and (2) reduced regulation of prices.

Greater Private-Sector Involvement

As discussed in previous chapters, the private health care sector plays an important role in India in spite of concerns about the quality of care it provides. In China, despite heightened interest in investing in health care services, private providers and hospitals still face many governmental restrictions; therefore, they often compete in the public sector under unequal conditions. We recommend that the Chinese government encourage both foreign and domestic investment in the private health care sector and that it provide a fair yet structured policy environment to nurture that sector's growth.

Reduced Regulation of Drug and Procedure Prices

Compared with India's free market economy, the Chinese government's decision to regulate prices has generated numerous problems. In particular, the overutilization of newly marketed drugs and expensive procedures is a very substantial issue that raises concerns about quality of care and financial burdens on the patient. For instance, the recent execution of the former head of the Chinese Food and Drug Administration, who accepted large bribes in return for approving faulty medicines, reveals the tip of the iceberg that is the disordered drug-approval procedure. We suggest that the government focus on regulating the quality, rather than the price, of drugs.

What Can India Learn from China?

Although India's health system was ranked higher than China's by WHO in 2000, Indian health is far poorer. The recent history of the Chinese health care system offers two particular lessons for Indian health policymakers: (1) increased spending on health and (2) better control of communicable diseases and improvements in maternal and infant health.

Increased Spending on Health, Especially Infrastructure, Providers, and Basic Necessities

Compared with China's government, the government of India contributes too little to health care, and the basic national health infrastructure, which includes clinics and preventive care services, lags behind. We suggest that the government make health care its top priority and allocate more resources at the village level.

Better Control of Communicable Diseases and Improvements in Maternal and Infant Health

A high proportion of deaths in India result from preventable causes. China outperforms India on almost all health indicators, especially birth outcomes and the control of communicable diseases. To show similar results, India's government must commit more resources to preventive and basic health care and coordinate efforts to improve hygiene, water quality, nutrition, and education and to reduce poverty reduction.

Conclusions

China and India are home to nearly two-fifths of the world population. Therefore, the challenges they face and the progress they make toward reforming their health systems are watched with close attention around the world. Lessons learned from China and India during the past three decades, combined with the effectiveness of the strategies these two countries adopt, will not only affect people who live in those two countries; they will also shed light on the needs and challenges of others.

Bibliography

Akin J. S., W. H. Dow, and M. Lance, "Changes in Access to Health Care in China, 1989–1997," *Health Policy and Planning*, Vol. 20, No. 2, March 2005, pp. 80–89.

Anderson, G. M., "Making Sense of Rising Caesarean Section Rates," *British Medical Journal*, Vol. 329, September 2004, pp. 696–697.

Barnum, H., J. Kutzin, and H. Saxenian, "Incentives and Provider Payment Methods," *International Journal of Health Planning and Management*, Vol. 10, No. 1, January–March 1995, pp. 23–45.

Beck, E. J., and N. Mays, "Health Care Systems in Transition III: The Indian Subcontinent," *Journal of Public Health Medicine*, Vol. 22, No. 1, March 2000, pp. 3–4.

Berman, P., "Rethinking Health Care Systems: Private Health Care Provision in India," *World Development*, Vol. 26, No. 8, August 1998, pp. 1,463–1,479.

Bhat, R., "Regulating the Private Health Care Sector: The Case of the Indian Consumer Protection Act," *Health Policy and Planning*, Vol. 11, No. 3, September 1996, pp. 265–279.

———, "Characteristics of Private Medical Practice in India: A Provider Perspective," *Health Policy and Planning*, Vol. 14, No. 1, March 1999, pp. 26–37.

Bhatia, J., and J. Cleland, "Health Care of Female Outpatients in South-Central India: Comparing Public and Private Sector Provision," *Health Policy and Planning*, Vol. 19, No. 6, November 2004, pp. 402–409.

Bloom, G., and X. Gu, "Health Sector Reform: Lessons from China," *Social Science & Medicine*, Vol. 45, No. 3, August 1997, pp. 351–360.

Bloom, G., L. Han, and X. Li, "How Health Workers Earn a Living in China," Sussex, U.K.: Institute of Development Studies, 2000.

Blumenthal, D., and W. Hsiao, "Privatization and Its Discontents—The Evolving Chinese Health Care System," *New England Journal of Medicine,* Vol. 353, No. 11, September 2005, pp. 1,165–1,170.

Cai, R. H., *China's Medical Security Reform*, Beijing: China Personnel Press, 1998.

The Central Party Committee and the State Council of China, *Decisions on Health Sector Reform and Development*, Beijing: The Central Party Committee and the State Council of China, 1997.

Chinese Ministry of Labor and Social Security, *Statistical Communication on Labor and Social Security Development in 2003*, Beijing, China: n.p., 2004.

Chinese Ministry of Health, *A Report on the National Health Services Survey in 1993*, Beijing: Ministry of Health, 1994.

———, *Health Statistics in China for 1995*, China: Ministry of Health, 1995.

———, *National Health Services Survey in 2003*, China: n.p., n.d. [2003].

———, *Zhongguo Weisheng Nianjian, 2004* [*China Health Year Book, 2004*], Beijing: People's Medical Publishing Company, 2004.

Chou, Y. J., W. Yip, C. Lee, N. Huang, Y. Sun, and H. Chang, "Impact of Separating Drug Prescribing and Dispensing on Provider Behavior: Taiwan's Experience," *Health Policy and Planning*, Vol. 18, No. 3, September 2003, pp. 316–329.

Das Gupta, M., and M. Rani, "India's Public Health System: How Well Does It Function at the National Level?" World Bank, Policy Research Working Paper No. 3447, November 1, 2004. As of May 2, 2008: http://econ.worldbank.org/external/default/main?pagePK=64165259&piPK=64165421&theSitePK=469372&menuPK=64216926&entityID=000012009_20041130093207

Datar, A., A. Mukherji, and N. Sood, "Health Infrastructure and Immunization Coverage in Rural India," *Indian Journal of Medical Research*, Vol. 125, No. 1, January 2007, pp. 31–42.

De Costa, A., and V. Diwan, "Where Is the Public Health Sector? Public and Private Sector Healthcare Provision in Madhya Pradesh, India," *Health Policy*, Vol. 84, No. 2–3, December 2007, pp. 269–276.

Devadasan, N., M. Boelaert, B. Criel, W. Van Damme, and B. Gryseels, "The Need for Strong General Health Services in India and Elsewhere," *Lancet*, Vol. 369, No. 9,562, February 2007, pp. 638–639.

Devadasan, N., B. Criel, W. Van Damme, K. Ranson, and P. Van der Stuyft, "Indian Community Health Insurance Schemes Provide Partial Protection Against Catastrophic Health Expenditure," *BioMed Central Health Services Research*, Vol. 7, No. 43, March 2007.

Devadasan, N., K. Ranson, W. Van Damme, A. Acharya, and B. Criel, "The Landscape of Community Health Insurance in India: An Overview Based on 10 Case Studies," *Health Policy*, Vol. 78, No. 2–3, October 2006, pp. 224–234.

Devadasan, N., and W. Van Damme, "Payments for Health Care in India," *Lancet*, Vol. 368, No. 9,554, December 2006, p. 2,209.

Drechsler, D., and J. P. Jütting, "Private Health Insurance in Low and Middle-Income Countries: Scope, Limitations, and Policy Responses," Issy-les-Moulineaux, France: Organisation for Economic Co-operation and Development, 2005.

Dror, D. M., R. Koren, A. Ost, E. Binnendijk, S. Vellakkal, and M. Danis, "Health Insurance Benefit Packages Prioritized by Low-Income Clients in India: Three Criteria to Estimate Effectiveness of Choice," *Social Science & Medicine*, Vol. 64, No. 4, February 2007, pp. 884–896.

Dror, D. M., R. Radermacher, and R. Koren, "Willingness to Pay for Health Insurance Among Rural and Poor Persons: Field Evidence from Seven Micro Health Insurance Units in India," *Health Policy*, Vol. 82, No. 1, July 2007, pp. 12–27.

Eggleston, K., and W. Yip, "Hospital Competition Under Regulated Prices: Application to Urban Health Sector Reforms in China" *International Journal of Health Care Finance and Economics*, Vol. 4, No. 4, December 2004, pp. 343–368.

Ensor, T., "Informal Payments for Health Care in Transition Economies," *Social Science & Medicine*, Vol. 58, No. 2, January 2004, pp. 237–246.

Government of India, *Report of the Health Survey and Development Committee*, Vol. II, Delhi: Manager of Publications, 1946.

Gupte, D. M., V. Ramachandran, and R. K. Mutatkar, "Epidemiological Profile of India: Historical and Contemporary Perspectives," *Journal of Biosciences*, Vol. 26, No. 4, November 2001, pp. 437–464.

Hanson K., W. Yip, and W. C. Hsiao, "Patients' Choice of Public and Private Providers in Cyprus: Implications for Price and Quality Competitions," *Health Economics*, Vol. 13, 2004, pp. 1,157–1,180.

Hesketh, T., and X. Z. Wei, "Health in China: From Mao to Market Reform," *British Medical Journal*, Vol. 314, May 1997, pp. 1,543–1,545.

Hesketh, T., and W. Zhu, "Health in China: The Healthcare Market," *British Medical Journal*, Vol. 314, May 1997, pp. 1,616–1,618.

Hsiao, W. C., "The Chinese Health Care System: Lessons for Other Nations," *Social Science & Medicine*, Vol. 41, No. 8, October 1995, pp. 1,047–1,055.

———, "Unmet Needs of Two Billion: Is Community Financing a Solution?" Health, Nutrition and Population Discussion Paper, Washington, D.C.: International Bank for Reconstruction and Development and World Bank, 2001.

———, "What is a Health System? Why Should We Care?" Harvard School of Public Health, August 2003. As of May 2, 3008:
www.hsph.harvard.edu/phcf/Papers/What%20Is%20A%20Health%20System-Final%20(general%20format)%208.5.03.pdf

———, "Why is a Systemic View of Health Financing Necessary?" *Health Affairs*, Vol. 26, No. 4, July–August 2007, pp. 950–961.

Hsiao, W. C., and P. S. Heller, *What Macroeconomists Should Know About Health Care Policy*, Washington, D.C.: International Monetary Find, 2007.

Hsiao, W. C., and Y. Liu, "Economic Reform and Health—Lessons from China," *New England Journal of Medicine*, Vol. 335, 2006, pp. 430–432.

Hsiao, W. C., and P. Shaw, *Social Health Insurance for Developing Nations*, Washington, D.C.: World Bank, 2007.

Huang, J., Y. Xue, Y. Jia, and J. Xue, "Evaluation of a Health Education Programme in China to Increase Breast-Feeding Rates," *Health Promotion International*, Vol. 9, No. 2, June 1994, pp. 95–98.

Koplan, J., L. Xingzhu, and L. Haichao, *Public Health in China: Organization, Financing and Delivery of Services*, World Bank working paper, July 2005.

Krishna, A., "Escaping Poverty and Becoming Poor: Who Gains, Who Loses, and Why?" *World Development*, Vol. 32, No. 1, January 2004, pp. 121–136.

Lee, D., and D. Yi, "A Novel Therapy for China: HMOs," *Los Angeles Times*, June 25, 2006, C1.

Lewis, M., "Informal Payments and the Financing of Health Care in Developing and Transition Countries," *Health Affairs*, Vol. 26, No. 4, 2007, pp. 984–997.

Lim, L., "The High Price of Illness in China," *BBC News*, Beijing, March 2, 2006.

Lim, M. K., H. Yang, T. Zhang, W. Feng, and Z. Zhou, "Public Perceptions of Private Health Care in Socialist China," *Health Affairs,* Vol. 23, No. 6, November–December 2004, pp. 222–234.

Lim, M. K., H. Yang, T. Zhang, Z. Zhou, W. Feng, and Y. Chen, "China's Evolving Health Care Market: How Doctors Feel and What They Think," *Health Policy*, Vol. 69, No. 3, September 2004, pp. 329–337.

Lipson R., "Investing in China's Hospitals," *The China Business Review*, Vol. 31, No. 6, 2004.

Liu, M., and X. Lu, "Health Care Quality Management in China Hospitals," in *Proceedings of the 2000 IEEE International Conference on the Management of Innovation and Technology*, Vol. 1, 2000, pp. 196–202.

Liu, X., and A. Mills, "The Effect of Performance-Related Pay of Hospital Doctors on Hospital Behaviour: A Case Study from Shandong, China," *Human Resources for Health*, Vol. 3, October 2005, p. 11.

Liu, Y., "China's Public Health-Care System: Facing the Challenges," *Bull World Health Organization*, Vol. 82, 2004, pp. 532–538.

Liu, Y., P. Berman, W. Yip, H. Liang, Q. Meng, J. Qu, and Z. Li, "Health Care in China: The Role of Non-Government Providers," *Health Policy*, Vol. 77, No. 2, July 2006, pp. 212–220.

Liu, Y., W. C. Hsiao, and K. Eggleston, "Equity in Health and Health Care: The Chinese Experience," *Social Science & Medicine*, Vol. 49, No. 10, November 1999, pp. 1,349–1,356.

Liu, Y., and K. Rao, "Providing Health Insurance in Rural China: From Research to Policy," *Journal of Health Politics, Policy and Law*, Vol. 31, No. 1, February 2006, pp. 71–92.

Liu, Y., K. Rao, and J. Fei, "Economic Transition and Health Transition: Comparing China and Russia," *Health Policy*, Vol. 44, May 1998, pp. 103–122.

Liu, Y., K. Rao, and W. C. Hsiao, "Medical Expenditure and Rural Impoverishment in China," *Journal of Health, Population, and Nutrition*, Vol. 21, No. 3, September 2003, pp. 216–222.

Mahal, A., "Health Policy Challenges for India—Private Health Insurance and Lessons from the International Experience," in T. N. Srinivasan, ed., *Trade, Finance and Investment in South Asia,* New Delhi: Social Science Press, 2002, pp. 417–476.

———, "Will Private Health Insurance Make the Distribution of Public Health Subsidies More Equal? The Case of India," *Geneva Papers on Risk and Insurance Theory,* Vol. 28, No. 2, December 2003, pp. 131–160.

Mahapatra, P., S. Srilatha, and P. Sridhar, "A Patient Satisfaction Survey in Public Hospitals," *Journal of the Academy of Hospital Administration,* Vol. 13., No. 2, 2001.

Markus, F., "China's Ailing Health Care," *BBC News,* Shanghai, December 7, 2004.

Mathur, S., "National Rural Health Mission—India," May 9, 2005. As of May 12, 2008:
http://www.pitt.edu/~super1/lecture/lec20541/001.htm

Meng, Q. Y., C. Gang, L. Silver, X. Sun, C. Rehnberg, and G. Tomson, "The Impact of China's Retail Drug Price Control Policy on Hospital Expenditures: A Case Study in Two Shandong Hospitals," *Health Policy and Planning,* Vol. 20, No. 3, 2005, pp. 185–196.

Mills, A., R. Brugha, K. Hanson, and B. McPake, "What Can Be Done About the Private Health Sector in Low-Income Countries?" *Bulletin of the World Health Organization,* Vol. 80, No. 4, April 2002, pp. 325–330.

Mullan, F., "Doctors For the World: Indian Physician Emigration," *Health Affairs,* Vol. 25, No. 2, March–April 2006, pp. 380–393.

National Bureau of Statistics of China, *China Statistical Yearbook,* Beijing, China: China Statistics Press, 2003.

———, *Statistical Communication on the 2003 National Economic and Social Development, Beijing,* China: n.p., 2004.

Pauly, M. V., P. Zweifel, R. M. Scheffler, A. S. Preker, and M. Bassett, "Private Health Insurance in Developing Countries," *Health Affairs,* Vol. 25, No. 2, March–April 2006, pp. 369–379.

Peters, D. H., K. S. Rao, and R. Fryatt, "Lumping and Splitting: The Health Policy Agenda in India," *Health Policy and Planning,* Vol. 18, No. 3, September 2003, pp. 249–260.

Peters, D. H., A. Wagstaff, L. Pritchett, N. V. Ramana, and R. R. Sharma, "Better Health Systems for India's Poor: Findings, Analysis, and Options," New Delhi: World Bank Publications, 2002.

Population Reference Bureau, *2006 World Population Data Sheet,* 2006. As of May 30, 2008:
http://www.prb.org/pdf06/06WorldDataSheet.pdf.

Project Team of the Development Research Center of the State Council of China, "An Evaluation of and Recommendations on the Reforms of the Health System in China," *China Development Review,* Vol. 7, No. 1, March 2005, supplement.

Purohit, B. C., "Private Initiatives and Policy Options: Recent Health System Experience in India," *Health Policy and Planning,* Vol. 16, No. 1, March 2001, pp. 87–97.

Qadeer, I., "Health Care Systems in Transition III: India, Part I. The Indian Experience," *Journal of Public Health Medicine,* Vol. 22, No. 1, March 2000, pp. 25–32.

Ramani, K. V., and M. Dileep, "Health System in India: Opportunities and Challenges for Improvements," Indian Institute of Management, July 2005.

Ramani, K. V., and D. Mavalankar, "Health System in India: Opportunities and Challenges for Improvements," *Journal of Health, Organisation and Management,* Vol. 20, No. 6, 2006, pp. 560–572.

Roberts, M. J., W. Hsiao, P. Berman, and M. R. Reich, *Getting Health Reform Right: A Guide to Improving Performance and Equity,* New York: Oxford University Press, 2004.

Roy, K., and D. H. Howard, "Equity in Out-of-Pocket Payments for Hospital Care: Evidence from India," *Health Policy,* Vol. 80, No. 2, February 2007, pp. 297–307.

Savedoff, W. D., "What Should a Country Spend on Health Care?" *Health Affairs,* Vol. 26, No. 4, July–August 2007, pp. 962–970.

Schneider, F., and D. Enste, *The Shadow Economy: Theoretical Approaches, Empirical Studies, and Political Implications*, Cambridge, U.K.: Cambridge University Press, 2002.

Sekhri, N., and W. Savedoff, "Private Health Insurance: Implications for Developing Countries," *Bulletin of the World Health Organization*, Vol. 83, No. 2, February 2005, pp. 127–138.

Selvaraju, V., "Public Expenditures on Health in India," background paper for the National Council of Applied Economic Research, 2000.

Sharma, M., "Health Education in India: A Strengths, Weaknesses, Opportunities, and Threats (SWOT) Analysis," *The International Electronic Journal of Health Education*, Vol. 8, 2005, pp. 80–85.

Shi, L., "Access to Care in Post-Economic Reform Rural China: Results from a 1994 Cross-Sectional Survey," *Journal of Public Health Policy*, Vol. 17, No. 3, 1996, pp. 347–361.

The State Council of China, *Decisions on Establishing the Basic Medical Insurance System for Urban Workers*, Beijing: The State Council of China, 1998.

Tang, K. C., D. Nutbeam, L. Kong, R. Want, and J. Yan, "Building Capacity for Health Promotion—A Case Study from China," *Health Promotion International*, Vol. 20, No. 3, September 2005, pp. 285–295.

United Nations in China, "China's Population: The Increasing Proportion of Elderly People," United Nations in China Web page, n.d. As of May 12, 2008:
http://www.unchina.org/about_china/html/population.shtml

Varatharajan, D., R. Thankappan, and J. Sabeena, "Assessing the Performance of Primary Health Centres Under Decentralized Government in Kerala, India," *Health Policy and Planning*, Vol. 9, No. 1, January 2004, pp. 41–51.

Wagstaff, A. N., N. Watanabe, and E. van Doorslaer, "Impoverishment, Insurance, and Health Care Payments," Health, Nutrition, and Population Discussion Paper, Washington, D.C.: World Bank, 2001.

Wang, H., J. Sindelar, and S. Busch, "The Impact of Tobacco Expenditure on Household Consumption Patterns in Rural China," *Social Science & Medicine*, Vol. 62, No. 6, March 2006, pp. 1,414–1,426.

Wang, H., W. Yip, L. Zhang, L. Wang, and W. Hsiao, "Community-Based Health Insurance in Poor Rural China: The Distribution of Net Benefits," *Health Policy and Planning*, Vol. 20, No. 6, November 2005, pp. 365–374.

Wang, H., L. Zhang, and W. C. Hsiao, "Ill Health and Its Potential Influence on Household Consumptions in Rural China," *Health Policy*, Vol. 78, October 2006, pp. 167–177.

Wang, H., L. Zhang, W. Yip, and W. Hsiao, "Adverse Selection in a Voluntary-Based Rural Mutual Health Care Insurance Scheme in Rural China," *Social Science & Medicine*, Vol. 63, No. 5, September 2006, pp. 1,236–1,245.

Whitehead, M., G. Dahlgren, and T. Evans, "Equity and Health Sector Reforms: Can Low-Income Countries Escape the Medical Poverty Trap?" *The Lancet*, Vol. 358, No. 9,284, September 2001, pp. 833–836.

WHO—*see* World Health Organization.

Wild, S., G. Roglic, A. Green, R. Sicree, and H. King, "Global Prevalence of Diabetes: Estimates for the Year 2000 and Projections for 2030," *Diabetes Care*, Vol. 27, No. 5, May 2004, pp. 1,047–1,053.

World Bank, *Financing Health Care: Issues and Options for China*, Washington, D.C.: World Bank, 1997.

———, "China's Rural Health Work: Multiple Challenges," n.p., 2004.

World Health Organization, *The World Health Report 2000—Health Systems: Improving Performance*, Geneva: World Health Organization, 2000.

———, "Death and DALY Estimates for 2002 by Cause for WHO Member States," spreadsheet, December 2004. As of May 30, 2008:
http://www.who.int/healthinfo/bod/en/index.html

———, *The World Health Report 2006: Working Together for Health*, Geneva: World Health Organization, 2006.

World Health Organization and the United Nations Children's Fund, *Primary Health Care: Report on the International Conference on Primary Health Care, Alma Ata, USSR, 6–12 September, 1978*, Geneva: World Health Organization, 1978.

Xu, K., D. B. Evans, G. Carrin, A. M. Aguilar-Rivera, P. Musgrove, and T. Evans, "Protecting Households from Catastrophic Health Spending," *Health Affairs*, Vol. 26, No. 4, July–August 2007, pp. 972–983.

Yip, W., and K. Eggleston, "Provider Payment Reform in China: The Case of Hospital Reimbursement in Hainan Province," *Health Economics*, Vol. 10, No. 4, June 2001, pp. 325–339.

———, "Addressing Government and Market Failures with Payment Incentives: Hospital Reimbursement Reform in Hainan, China," *Social Science & Medicine*, Vol. 58, No. 2, January 2004, pp. 267–277.

Yip, W., and W. C. Hsiao, "Medical Savings Accounts: Lessons from the People's Republic of China," *Health Affairs*, November–December 1997, pp. 226–231.

Yip, W., and H. Wang, "Determinants of Patient Choice of Medical Providers: A Case Study in Rural China," *Journal of Health Policy and Planning*, Vol. 13, No. 3, September 1998, pp. 311–322.

Yu, Y., "Market Economy and Social Justice: The Predicament of the Underprivileged," *The Journal of Comparative Asian Development*, Vol. 5, No. 1, 2006.